Saying Goodbye to Sonny

by

Karen Rihn

DEDICATION

TO:
ALOYSIUS JR. (MY FATHER)
SONNY (ALOYSIUS 111)
GAIL (SONNY'S WIFE)
RICHARD RIHN (TOM'S BROTHER)
MARGARET RIHN (TOM'S MOTHER)
WEEZIE (MY SISTER)
MARY K. (MY MOTHER)
GERALD RIHN (TOM'S FATHER)
DONNA RIHN (TOM'S SISTER)

ALL IN OUR IMMEDIATE FAMILY WHO
HAVE GONE BEFORE US. GIVE US THE
ENERGY FROM ABOVE TO PROPEL US
THROUGH OUR LIVES.
SAVE ME A SPOT, SONNY. YOU
PROMISED!

**TO MY HUSBAND TOM; MY FORTRESS
AND MY GUIDING LIGHT.

CONTENTS

Prologue:

My mother often tells this story:

When Sonny was three years old , we were set to go to his cousin's birthday party. I was fussing around the house, picking up the whatnots left by the kids and the whole time Sonny was begging me to leave. I recognized his love for food; especially birthday cake was the reason for his restlessness. When I told him "No, the party doesn't start yet, it's not time." His reply was, "I'll go early to put out the poons."

CHAPTER 1

The Annunciation

It was one of those cold December Friday nights when Tom and I were settled in to simply relax after a hard week at work. Tom is a Professor in Pharmacy and has a continuing education consulting business. I am a Special Education teacher in an elementary school. Friday nights were a welcome invitation to just chill. I was anxiously awaiting "Providence", a weekly staple in my lineup of favorite TV shows when the phone rang. I expected to be discussing "Providence" with my sister, Weezie, who lived in Indianapolis. It never failed that one of us would call the other and get the stage set for this show about a family in Providence Rhode Island.

We enjoyed comparing the two sisters and their
relationship to us. "Who do you think Joanie
will fall in love this week? or "Can you believe
Sid!" She played a Physician who moved back
to her hometown to be close to her family.   It
was the wonderful, gossipy girl talk that sisters
love to share especially when it's about a
dysfunctional family that is not ours.

The phone call, however, was from my
brother Sonny, who lived in Chicago. He and his
wife Gail had lived in a small town outside of
Pittsburgh most of their lives. But when his
company, J&L Steel, where he was human
relations director became LTV he was forced to
move to Munster, Indiana also a small town just
west of Chicago.

J&L Steel was situated on the bank of the
Monongahela River in the Hazelwood section of
Pittsburgh. Molten steel was produced, then
hauled by train across the Hot Metal Bridge to
the J&L Southside Works rolling mills on the left
bank. After rolling and cooling, a portion of the
steel was brought back to Hazelwood where
some went through the finishing mills (mostly
wire and nails) and the rest went into the storage
buildings. Major structural steel was shipped
directly from the Southside Works. It was

Sonny's job to hire, and oversee to the needs of the 8,500 people employed. In 1968, LTV purchased J & L, and then merged with Republic Steel in 1985. One year later, Republic Steel was forced to close due to foreign competition, high labor costs, and a lack of modern steel-making equipment. Steel making became a thing of the past in Pittsburgh, leaving many without a job and necessitating a totally new career path.

"Hi Kitten, (his nickname for me), how ya doing? I'm just calling everybody to check in because I have to tell you all something." Everybody meant my other three brothers, sister, and my Mother. "I just had a checkup because I wasn't feeling good and they found that I might have Leukemia." Twas such a matter of fact statement that all I could do is day, "What?" Did I hear him right? Not my brother, not the strong one of this family, not someone so full of life. Only children get leukemia. My head became a beehive of horrible thoughts with his words.

A black sterile phone became the sole means to convey the plethora of emotions that followed. I was supportive by trying to come up with empty words and downplaying a disease of which I know nothing about other than that it could be deadly.

With Christmas very close, Sonny went on to outline his course for recovery. He explained he would enter the hospital at Northwestern in Chicago after Christmas and begin chemotherapy. Gail would drive him there and no one would be needed to help. We all might be contacted in the future to be tested for a bone marrow match, but that was not a certainty. Looking back, he must have practiced that phone call over and over to have been able to relay this message in such an orderly, logical fashion. Our conversation ended with my assurance of being there to help at any time and looking ahead to next Christmas when all this would be an unpleasant memory. Tears began to flow from both of us when we said our "love you's" followed by a click to abruptly end the call.

Tom remained quiet and attentive during our conversation. He was well aware of the potential severity of this diagnosis. As a brother-in-law, thoughts of the jovial good times they shared together immediately came to his mind. It never failed, when Sonny was involved there would be an abundance of laughter and antics. Sonny once promised to move our great aunt. He rounded up my other brothers and Tom to help that Saturday morning. Aunt Norma had some very delicate French provincial tables with long spindly legs.

Sure enough, in the U-Haul truck one of the legs broke off. Tom, being a bit of a perfectionist, was quite upset that this had happened. Sonny's reaction was, "Don't worry, I'll talk to her." Bad went to worse when a beveled glass mirror broke as my brothers Danny and Gilbert were carrying it up the narrow third floor steps to her apartment. They simply put it face down in the living room for her to discover later. The final blow happened when that delicate three-legged table was dropped to become leg-less. At that point it ended up in the woods behind the apartment. They all had the best intentions, helping their widowed old aunt, they were just not movers. Sonny's final comment, as he shook his head and held his chin was "I'll have to talk to her." All three erupted in irrepressible laughter realizing that there was no foreseeable good outcome other than exhaustion. Fortunately, about three fourths of the way into the move, they found two teenager fellows and paid them to finish. Ever since, this group is referred to as "Ace Movers" but they spell it "Ass".

You can only imagine the chain of phone calls that followed that December night. My brothers Danny, Pierce, and Gilbert to me, I to my mother, all in disbelief, but hopeful and faithful that this disease can be beat. The final phone call was from Weezie. We didn't discuss "Providence", we just cried together.

CHAPTER 2

The Visit

We celebrated Christmas that year as robots going through the actions but really wanting to surround our brother with non-stop love and nurturing. Everyone stayed in touch and with each phone call Sonny assured us he and Gail were fine together for the holiday and he was anxious to get on with the treatment in Chicago. He would even joke with my mom and say, "Chubby, (his nickname for her) don't eat too much ham or we'll need a crane to get you out of that chair." He constantly made my mother laugh with his visits. Always his big fat face smile ready to listen to our woes but never willing to share any of his. However, this year, the weather was as cold and bleak as the feelings in our hearts. It is the limbo time that holds one captive in a state of uncertainty and unstably regret of the present.

Mid-January came and my relentless desire to be with Sonny was finally at hand. Sonny's unremitting offers to show off Chicago were meaningless in the present situation. There will be the next trip when you can showcase all your favorite spots, but for now it's all about you, I thought as I boarded USAir on a Friday after school. I began my adventure on the first weekend of his chemo at Northwestern University Hospital. After planes, trains, and taxis, I arrived to see him in his hospital bed with a wide smile on his fat face surprised to see me. Already he had won the hearts of every nurse as he proudly introduced his baby sister. The chemo had been started and his long waiting game had begun.

During the afternoon, Sonny and I reminisced about the funny times we shared growing up in a family of six kids. I reminded him of the time Mom and Dad came screaming up to his bedroom ranting about his actions the night before. My brothers and sister were all startled by the commotion so early on a Saturday morning. It turns out that Sonny had told my parents he was going to see Gail, his girlfriend at the time. They assumed Sonny would simply walk up the street to Gail's sister, Jill's house. However Gail's parents lived an hour and a half away up in the mountains of Ligonier. They somehow never imagined that Sonny would venture out on a frigid winter night to make the trip to Gail's parents! Since the roads to Ligonier would be far too treacherous, my parents would have never given their approval.

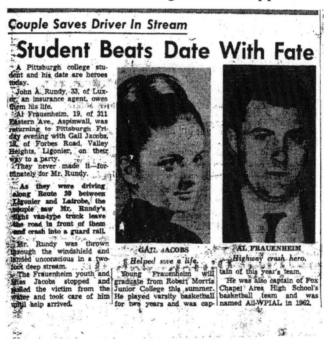

Couple Saves Driver In Stream

Student Beats Date With Fate

A Pittsburgh college student and his date are heroes today.

John A. Rundy, 33, of Luxor, an insurance agent, owes them his life.

Al Frauenheim, 19, of 311 Eastern Ave., Aspinwall, was returning to Pittsburgh Friday evening with Gail Jacobs, 18, of Forbes Road, Valley Heights, Ligonier, on their way to a party.

They never made it—fortunately for Mr. Rundy.

As they were driving along Route 30 between Ligonier and Latrobe, the couple saw Mr. Rundy's light van-type truck leave the road in front of them and crash into a guard rail.

Mr. Rundy was thrown through the windshield and landed unconscious in a two-foot deep stream.

The Frauenheim youth and Miss Jacobs stopped and pulled the victim from the water and took care of him until help arrived.

GAIL JACOBS
Helped save a life.

Young Frauenheim will graduate from Robert Morris Junior College this summer. He played varsity basketball for two years and was cap-

AL FRAUENHEIM
Highway crash hero.

tain of this year's team. He was also captain of Fox Chapel Area High School's basketball team and was named All-WPIAL in 1962.

As my parents were having their morning coffee they heard on the news about a courageous rescue made for a man whose car had landed in

Ligonier Creek. The headlines read: "Student Beats Date With Fate" and

"Couple Saves Driver in Stream". The hero was a boy named Al Frauenheim which is Sonny's real name. Looking back, that explosion coming from my parents was their realization that it could have been him in the creek with no one to bring them to safety. The "hero" was grounded for one month.

I was content to sit by his bedside for the duration of my time with him, but he had other plans! "Kitten, you have to try a Ghirardelli milkshake on Michigan Avenue. Go out turn left, and then follow Michigan to the Water Tower. It's right on the corner. While you're there go in Filene's Basement. You'll love the shopping. I followed his orders as I always have and was delightfully surprised and enchanted with the city of Chicago. The bustling city with people smiling, chatting , scurrying to find the next item on their agendas were out of place considering my perspective. I followed his orders and walked through Barnes and Nobel to pick up some sports magazines for him, went two doors down to Ghirardelli's to get a little lunch at an adjacent French café, then ordered a takeout.

We were raised on chocolate sodas and milkshakes! My mother used them as a remedy for all sickness, somewhat like antibiotics today. She always defended her ways by blaming them on the fact that her Father, Grandpa Brown, had owned and been the Pharmacist at a prominent Drug Store in downtown Pittsburgh. Years ago before CVS and Walgreens, drug stores typically had a huge fountain area front and center in the stores which served hand scooped ice cream of all flavors. A fountain person was hired to man the job of serving the customers delicious drinks and sundaes. My Mother spent many a summer working at Grandpa Brown's drug store. She learned to scoop out delicious flavors into a stainless steel container, pump chocolate syrup, add whole milk, then whip it all up under a thin spindle until a flawless milkshake had been created.

Ghirardelli chocolate milkshake , the perfect pick-me-up for Sonny when he's faced with eating the hospital dinner for the evening, enveloped my mind and catapulted me back to the hospital.

I found Sonny in the special waiting room with his IV connected. It was a sad contrast, sitting in that room when just outside the windows the exciting city loomed. The other patients, many hairless as a result of the chemo portrayed a glum predictor of the months to come. As I happily pulled out the ultimate "cure" which he whisked out of my hand and took two sips of before handing it back to keep for later; definitely not typical for my brother or any of us.

Again, Sonny got "antsy" for me and sent me on my way to the Cathedral for Mass at 5:00, then dinner. I found the glorious church named St. Louis Cathedral in the daylight and immediately thought it was everything as spectacular as Sonny had described. The setting sunlight sliced through stained glass which lined the church. The altar stood ethereally up high as if God would appear at any moment. As in many situations for me, my emotional guards broke down. Tears streamed down my face. I didn't cry for Sonny's disease because I found comfort in the fact that his treatment was started at a renowned hospital and the healing process was in place. My tears came because he wasn't here to experience this divine moment with me and because I had waited too long to visit as he had wanted, so he could show off his beloved Cathedral.

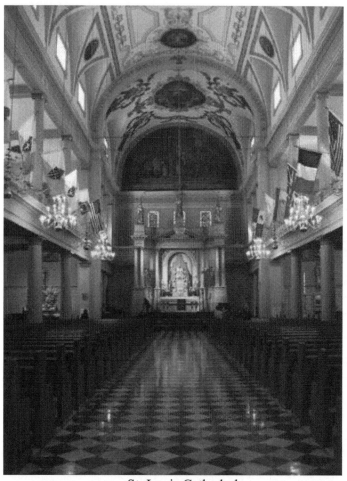

St. Louis Cathedral

After Mass, navigating back in a strange dark city turned out to be a definite challenge if not impossible to remember and recognize the landmarks that all looked the same in each passing shadow. My body manuvered through groups of unknown people; eyes down, bulldozing along the streets with no names. Leave it to Sonny to put me in a fix like this. The situation brought to my mind a flash back. As one of six children, I "luckily" was left to find my own entertainment. One Saturday of my 14th year, Sonny asked me to come along with he and Gail to ski at a Ski Lodge named 7 Springs about an hour from Pittsburgh. Since I had never been to 7 Springs or skied before, the excitement took over my whole being. As Mom and Dad easily gave their approval since I would be with my Big Brother, I was setting myself up for the time of my life!!! - and it was. We successfully learned to rent the equipment. However I had to buckle Sonny's boots since he couldn't bend over far enough to latch them. We skied down the beginner's hill outside the lodge, and even ventured up our first chair lift. What a feeling, to fly through the crisp biting air over the snow covered tree tops to eventually be dropped off at the top of the mountain! I mean dropped off literally! Sonny plummeted from the chair, sliding down the ramp with both skies dandling attached to his feet only by the boot straps. Gail and I were much more graceful as we exited our first chair lift ride. Laughter erupted from everywhere around us as onlookers took in this sight.

I especially remember how yummy that first bite of the prefixed dinner tasted after we stood in a line that stretched through the entire lobby. I was over the top in love with this experience. After dinner we met a group of Sonny's friends in the Matterhorn, a bar in the lodge. Gail was a cute cheerleader and Sonny was the captain of the basketball team so needless to say they were in the popular group for their Senior year of high school . As the evening progressed I may have had a sip or two of beer, because we were in a bar, but the real fun was the dancing and joking around. I even got to meet a guy whom Sonny introduced as Nat the Rat. As a fourteen year old, I remember him as being extremely tall and skinny. I think because he must have felt sorry for Sonny's tag along little sister, he asked me to swing dance. He swung me all over the place, including the top of the bar. Didn't someone take a picture of us which landed smack dab on the front page of the 7 Spring's Newsletter and my parents' breakfast table. So much for being safe with my Big Brother!

When Northwestern Hospital finally came into site my fears immediately diminished. It was home for me that weekend, but it was Sonny's home for the next 3 painful months. As I checked on Sonny for the last time, I found him sleeping with the IV attached and the milkshake on his bed stand, untouched.

CHAPTER 3

Realization

What is leukemia? I could delve into a scientific explanation to answer this question with a click onto Google. Information comes flying to us in many forms today. We are socially and intellectually connected at the blink of an eye. But neither I nor my siblings were ready to be emotionally connected to the details of leukemia. They orbited around our heads like little planets that were not going to come crashing in on our Sun! We chose the splintered paths of speculation, rather than hard facts of science. "What do you think?" my brother Gil would ask, "Does he have the acute myeloid leukemia or the other kind?" The answer coming from someone who has a husband with a Doctor of Pharmacy and two sons attending medical school was always, "I don't know."

But I did know:

Chronic Myeloid Leukemia is one of the four major types of leukemia that is treated daily with oral drug therapy. Most patients are diagnosed during CML's chronic phase when symptoms are mild or not noticeable. During this phase, your white cells can still fight infection. In most cases, long-term drug therapy can control chronic phase CML, and you can usually return to normal activities after treatment begins. A small number of people diagnosed and treated during the chronic phase progress to the accelerated phase when the patient no longer responds to the medication.

The chances of survival are good with close monitoring by a hematologist or oncologist.

Acute Myeloid Leukemia is another major type. Acute myeloid leukemia (AML) is a cancer of the bone marrow and the blood that progresses quickly without treatment. It affects mostly cells that aren't fully developed. These cells can't carry out their normal functions. That's one reason why it's important to get care and treatment as soon as possible.

One clue to which type Sonny was diagnosed with was the quickness in beginning his treatment. ASAP were the directives Sonny was told by his oncologist. Potent chemotherapy drugs were given to put his leukemia cells into remission. These drugs also affect normal cells sometimes causing a multitude of side effect.

One treatment used for AML patients after the chemotherapy is a bone marrow transplant. A bone marrow transplant allows the oncologist to aggressively treat the leukemia with chemotherapy which kills all the cells and then replace healthy bone marrow. All five of us were tested seeking a match and not one of us was a match.

Sonny's road was a slippery slide from the comfortable but inconvenient state I left him in. In the following months he developed a rash which enveloped his body and inside his mouth and throat. This condition, Steven's Johnson Syndrome, is an adverse reaction to the strong chemotherapy used in fighting the leukemic cells. He remained in the hospital for all of February and March. During that time my sister, Weezie, was able to visit often and give support to Gail who, herself, suffered from kidney disease. She kept those of us in Pittsburgh well-informed.

CHAPTER 4

SPRING

May came. Spring had arrived. The budding flowers and trees made their presence onto hightened senses that year. I was oblivious to the countdown of days left in the school year or the longer lit evenings that repalced the darkness of winter nights. Our joy came in the fact that Sonny had been released from the hospital and was going home to be with Gail in their little town of Munster Indiana. A place none of us had ever visited since Sonny had moved and lived for over four years. Time for my first visit!!!

Over a long weekend I flew into Chicago, took the train to an adjacent town where Gail was waiting to pick me up. Munster is a neat postage stamp town with sidewalks and houses surrounding a Main Street full of the independently owned stores that provide for the needs of its occupants; food, clothing, and shelter; just like Aspinwall the town we all grew up in.

In Aspinwall, we lived in one of those large old, 3 story victorian homes on a corner lot. Our front porch stretched across the the house and overlooked two treelined streets, which shielded anyone who might be sitting on it. Every night weather permitting, my parents would forego the usual TV and escape to sit, rock, and talk about things, especially about the people walking by who were unaware of our tree-hidden presence. None of us would come home for the night without slipping into the front porch conversations. I listened and took-in the accounts of all the adventures of the day and gossip of the poor unsuspecting passers by, until my blurry eyes and sleepy head told me it was time for bed. Looking back I realized this time was our bedtime story; not a personal tuck in by Mom and Dad, but intimate, sharing of our lives in the presence of each other.

Of course, no one could top Sonny's adventures. One late Fall evening my Dad was recapping the Halloween Sonny almost got arrested. He and my mother were in a line to see the family doctor that formed in the large room above our local burrough building/police station. Our Doctor serviced almost everyone in Aspinwall but never gave appointments. It was strictly first-come first-served on Monday and Thursday evenings, resulting in lines of patients waiting their perspective turn. As my Dad held his position in route, his eye caught a crowd of young teenage boys outside the window being pushed around and herded up by the local police. The violent activity angered my Dad to the point of him giving up his spot in line and confronting the police officers to question the reasons for their outrage. They reported that the boys had just played a number of Halloween pranks throughout the town and needed to be repremanded for their actions. My Father's outrage to the rough treatment grew with the recognition that it was Halloween and classic pranks were almost expected by this age group. As he looked around he noticed that the boys were all Sonny's friends, but Sonny was no where to be seen. After suggesting to the police to at least give a call to the kids' parents and let them handle the situation, he and my mother headed for the 5 block walk home. As they approached the front porch, there Sonny sat looking battered and sweaty from being out of breath. "Have a nice night?" said my Dad in a calm tone. "You bet! Jackie Babe and I were just running through the woods and I caught my pants on a bush. Can you sew them, Mom?" My Dad replied, "I just saw your friends down at the police station. They were getting a little roughed up. I told the police to call their parents and let them handle it. I'm glad your home . Now go to bed." Sonny obediently passed me by with a smile and a wink as he ascended to his bedroom.

When entering the sweet 3 bedroom colonial house in Munster, I was greeted by "Hey Chubby". I guess I inherited my mother's nickname. Our arms enveloped each other with a hug lasting an eternity. I held my own and was proud that no tears were shed, just joy to be in their presence. However, half of Sonny was gone. His 220 pound tank of a body had became a frail 150. His fat rounded face was reduced to sunken cheeks and gray eyes. Gail immediately busied herself by preparing a lunch of sandwiches and iced tea while Sonny and I talked. Not about him, his sickness, or his hellish ordeal, but about my kids, Tom, my mother, the

Aspinwall news. Just like the riviting old front porch conversations. It was good to be there!!! That night I slept on the sofa in the living room that banked up against a window. The light from the streetlamp streamed in creating a path for my multitude of thoughts and prayers to venture out. Being lost in this light, watching the back and forth movement of the gold laden clock Sonny was given for his retirement from LTV, and feeling the closeness of my dieing brother, gave a sleepless night to cherish forever.

The next morning exploded into the arrival of my sister, Weezie. Since she lived in Indianapolis she was able to drive in and visit often. Weezie was larger than life, always laughing and kidding. Years ago as children we were all playing in Aspinwall's community park where football games were played on Friday nights. Parents, (in the old days) would simply let the kids go out and play. We would leave the house after breakfast and sometimes not come back till dinner. There were no cell phones or Nannies to ease a parent's concern on the well being of their children throughout the day. Life, especially in summer time was left to the kids banding together and creating their own fun. However, red flags went up and phones started buzzing if by any chance you didn't show up in time for dinner. To this day I feel an urgency to be home by the dinner hour and my children haven't lived at home for years.

Well, as we all played in the park that day, Weezie felt adventurous and climbed the goal post on the football field. One by one she drew an audience of concerned kids warning to jump or not to jump after being stuck at the top middle crossbar of the post. All heads and eyes were focused upward to see what Weezie was going to do, when a voice from a house on the adjacent street yelled, "Stay put, I just called the police." Sure enough within the next minute we heard the piercing sirens of the fire department and police cars competing to save my sister. The full search and rescue instantly was orchestrated by our small town with competent emergency services. Needless to say, there was quite a story retold around the dinner tables that night in Aspinwall!

That morning Weezie's robust nature got us all up and moving. "I'm here to help. What can we do?" Of cource Sonny protested but in his weakened state and knowing that Gail was not strong enough for yard work and heavy cleaning, he put us to work! First order of business was to buy some flowers to make the yard more cheerful and Spring-like. That was my idea. Being with Weezie was an ongoing party, even if only a trip to Kmart. We got all the chitchat and concerns out of the way in the car so we could consentrate on giving Sonny and Gail a respite from the months before. Sonny became the bedridden director for us to mow the lawn and find the necessary tools for planting and gardening. Mutt and Jeff would have been too kind of a nickname for the manner that Weezie and I approached our tasks. "How do you start this mower? "Where did you say the shovel is?" " Does your yard go all the way back to the fence?" Sonny often used an expression of frustation with us. It was the sing of the cross in Latin.

In nomine(pr. nomeen) patris, et filii(pr. filee), et spiritus sanctum Amen. Sonny finally bounded down the steps and out the backdoor to answer our questions and get the mower started. We were finally busy at work trying to finish before nightfall. As the evening came we all were giddy as we languidly sat on the back porch to recap the day. The entire time a wave of feelings swept over me. In this midst of the horrible disease Sonny had to deal with, we were able to manifest our usual heartfelt love for each other by doing what was needed and supressing our sullen feelings into fun-loving memories.

As I started for my exit the next morning, the vision of the backyard caught my eye and still remains fixed. The yard with dew-laden fresh cut grass and sprays of virgin flowers cast a fresh Spring-like vision of new life, hope, dreams that things will stay constant; not better but just like the moment at hand. The visit was over. I plopped down on a window seat of the airplane bound for home and the tears began to flow all the way to Pittsburgh.

Chapter 5

Summer Vacation

June is a month that everyone looks forward to and enjoys! The children and teachers are out of school, many weddings and graduations take place with lavish celebrations. That June the break from the rigors of balancing schoolwork and family was a welcome and appeciated arrival after a winter and Spring of worry, frustration, and uncertainty. I was attuned to the sweet wake up calls of the birds, the brightness and feel of the hot sun, the still moments caught latenight under the stars.

Tom's career in Pharmacy was three dimentional; always going in a multitude of directions and taking advantage of every opportunity that came his way. Many days at 7:00 he would leave to teach a class at Duquesne University, head over to his educational consulting company, then at 3:00 fly off to give a program to a group of pharmacists or doctors. His hard work made it possible for us to purchase a three bedroom beach townhouse in Ocean City, Maryland. This corner house sat at the edge of the Bay facing the west. The master bedroom stretched all across the front of the house leaving the two bedrooms along the backside. Each night the house was embraced by the most glorious sunsets! Everything stopped at this time as we toasted the dusk on the decks of the front porch or bedroom deck. On a cloudless night the sun's presence enveloped the bedroom as if it were about to make a direct landing. This is the bedroom Sonny and Gail had when they came for a visit in June.

Sonny and Gail had always enjoyed traveling and this year was no exception. They were delighted to revisit Ocean City; pointing out and remenising about the places they had stayed on previous trips. Up and down Coastal Highway Sonny would say, "Remember that place, Kitten, that's where we stayed with Mom and Dad. There's the place we had the best crab dinner!" He was like a little kid on Christmas when out and about, seeing the sights, and thinking about food. On their arrival Gail realized that they had forgotten a vital piece of equipment needed for medication delivery. This immediately brought them back to the real world of dealing with the disease. Gail took her role as caregiver very seriously and indelibly became deflated by this issue. Whereas Sonny turned the whole thing into a joke, "Hey Graham, my youngest son, go over to 7 Eleven and get a super gulp and I'll use the big straw to plug it up. Tom needed to stay in Pittsburgh with my son Andy's soccer tournament. They were due to come in a few days. But with his long distant guidance we found the necessary device at the local hospital.

The first night my brother Gil, his wife Ginny and their 15 year old son, Pierce arrived to stay the week. After a welcoming dinner and sunset ceremony, everyone was completely tuckered out, except Graham and Pierce. To 12 and 15 year olds, 9:00 was not the time things wound down in Ocean City. There was the boardwalk looming only 100 streets away! Teenagers found the allure of the food, games, shops eternally exciting. "Should we buy that leash with an invisible dog." " Let's play the rock star drum game." "Where are the fake tatoes?" "Oh, let's get some Thrashers French Fries!" After much debate, we allowed Graham to be intrusted to his cousin's care to take the bus to the boardwalk. The deal was set only if they would return on the 11:00 bus. Promises were quickly agreed on and they happily departed. At 11:00 the adults made the assent to bed. Sonny especially looked like he had spent all the energy he had for a day. I was sleeping on the couch which left me to hold vigil for our wayward boys. Every minute after 11:30 ticked like a timebomb in my head. No sign of the boys. Just as I began to scroung around for my shoes to drive to the bus stop, Sonny came barraling down the steps with his jacket on and fishing hat pulled down around his face. "We're going after them!" he muttered as he passed by to the nearest exit door. I could tell that he had been holding the vigil with me. He and I got in his car, he drove to the bus stop and luckily they were just getting off the bus at 11:45. A little late but safe and sound in Sonny's car. "The 11:00 bus was full." were the only words spoken for the rest of that night. Our presence was enough to send them the messages of concern, worry, and love.

The next day was spent in a mellifluous manner; easy, lazy living. Sonny could not really navigate the long sandy walk across the beach. Instead he enjoyed the crashing waves from the perimeter. Quite a contrast from years before of the daring human body surfer who professed no wave being too much; " for this tank of a body".

Later in the day we all took refuge at the pool to soak up the brilliant rays of the sun. The entire time as I lazed on a chase, my partially opened eyes, hidden by the darkness of sunglasses, witnessed Sonny trudging back and forth in the lap pool with his poor frail body and his fishing hat pulled down over his face. I can't help but think he was trying to walk off the leukemia like shedding unwanted pounds. To date my brother Gil and I have privately named that part of the pool, Sonny's lane.

Family reunions are sometimes planned and executed annually, but never in our family. As we all grew up, busy careers, distance, children's activities all acted as deterents to reuniting for more of the front porch exchanges we were so used to growing up. This summer was different. The beach house served as our family reunion that year for at least half of my family. Tom and Andy arrived for the weekend. Soon after, my brother Pierce, his wife Ann, and one of their seven children, Scott made a surprise one night visit from their home in New Jersey. My type C personality was unshaken by the additional company. The question of dinner was quickly solved by a trip to the local seafood carry out store where Pierce bought so much shrimp, crabs, clams, and lobster that he was given a hat

that bore the name of the restaurant! Pierce
proudly sported that hat the entire night. We had
a delightful evening beginning with the sunset
and ending late under a skyful of stars. Stories
were told and retold.

As much as our brother Sonny was the glue
of the family, Pierce is the star! In 1961 he was a
vital member of the Rutgers football team that
had an undefeated season, playing on both the
offense and defense teams. His picture was in
Time Magazine! Pierce was married to Ann
soon after college. They presently have seven
children, 19 grandchildren, and 3 great
grandchildren; most of which live within five
minutes of their home in New Jersey. Pierce
remained in a small town close to Rutgers and
accepted a position as Athletic
Director then football coach at a co-ed catholic
school called Immaculata. " Under Frauenheim,
the football program has won 4 state titles (25
State Play-off Berths) and 23 conference
championships, compiling an overall record of
313-132-2 ." He has been in this position for 50
years!

The road for him was not always easy. In
1974 he was diagnosed with cancer of the larnyx.
He had surgury which removed his voicebox.

How does a football coach with six children at the time, continue without a voice? His deep faith brought him the courage he needed to use a system called esophageal speaking: "air is injected into the upper esophagus and then released in a controlled manner to create sound used to produce speech. Esophageal speech is a learned skill that requires speech training and much practice." Pierce learned this system and was able to remain a constant leader in his position as a coach, a teacher, and a principal. He has secured many accolades in his career. Greg Gumball produced a documentary for the American Cancer Society showcasing his couragous journey. Each time I have been lucky enough to hear Pierce speak after receiving an award, I am amazed at his humility, faith and motivation. His response is always the same; "If I can do it so can you."   He is also currently a motivational speaker for football clinics, High School Assemblies and Corporations.

I don't know which I treasured the most. The fact that we were indeed sharing precious time together or that our kids were there to witness, hear, and experience first hand what family means. No one asked to go to the boardwalk that night!

Andy and Graham were kept quite busy checking on the stock market with Sonny. First thing Sonny would ask in the morning was , "O.K. man what's it at now?" They quickly learned to be on top of this issue and proudly spurted off the latest Dow and NASDAC numbers. 1999 was a year of wheeling and dealing in the stock market which thankfully took a bit of Sonny's attention away from the real issues at hand. This was their first introduction to any sort of business or money exchanges. Both Andy and Graham majored in business and are currently working in marketing and finance.

The final evening , after Pierce, Ann, and Scott had headed home, we decided to go out for dinner to a Maryland favorite, Phillips Crab House. This restaurant is located directly in the hubbub of the boardwalk. The victorian décor with enchanting chandilars and the cozy corner table we were seated at in the bar area made for an unforgettable time. Sonny and Gail had no children so they truly enjoyed the dining out experience. Every waiter or waitress lucky enough to serve them became their immediate sounding board and confidant. "Honey, two waters lots of ice, O.K.?" Sonny would spurtout.

By the time the dinner was served we had first hand details about the life of our waitress from Sonny's questions and interest. After dinner the young ones went off happily to explore boardwalk fun. That left the adults to linger and listen to the piano bar tunes of Britt and Apple, a duo performing for the evening. Tom and I decide to dance to a Frank Sinatra tune. Out of the corner of my eye I noticed that Gil and Ginny had joined us quickly followed by Sonny and Gail. All of us together dancing, who would have thought after the winter we had just come through. As a surprise to me, Tom secretly made a request which Apple slendidly sang. It was entitled "Sunny" by Bobby Hebb .

" Sunny, yesterday my life was filled with pain. Sunny, you smiled at me and really eased the pain. Oh the dark days are done , the bright days are here. My Sunny one shines so sincere. Sunny one so true Sunny I love you."
It was my pleasure to dance that one with guess who.

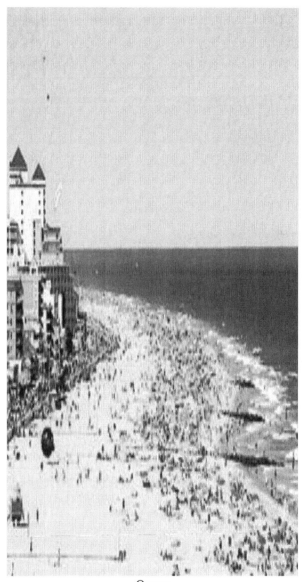

Ocean
City, MD

Chapter 6

Chicago Chicago

We live in an extremely territorial society. People from the East are particial to the East. When People from Pittsburgh talk big city we think New York or Philadelphia. For water vacations we think the shore, the beach, anywhere on the Atlantic Ocean. Unless you had a reason or were visiting a relative, it was not likely that a "Northeasterner" would venture to the middle of the country.

That is exactly how it happened that my family decided to take a weekend August trip and finally explore the city that Sonny had so often spoken of wanting to show off. As we all piled out of the car in Munster, Indiana I noticed something. Each of our four boys had put on the

Chicago Bulls hat that their Uncle Sonny at onetime or another given them. Even Tom sported a Bulls 1996 championship hat that Sonny had sent back in June. Sonny LOVED the Bulls and often called to offer tickets, especially to my older sons Chris and Jeff. The timing was never quite right for them each being in medical school. But the time was right now and we were set to have the first hand tour!

We all piled in Sonny's Lincoln, with Gail graciously staying behind to allow six of us to fit in the car. I suspected Gail welcomed a chance to be alone. Sonny was at the wheel with his fishing hat pulled down low and his tired body ably navigating through the streets of downtown Chicago. "East End Ave. that's where Oprah lives, I think", he happily shouted. We drove all through Michigan Avenue, saw the Chicago Sun Times Building, saw the Navy Pier, drove past the famous Art Museum, the Bears Stadium, swung around to where the University of Illinois which is preceded by the distinguished brown stones that house professors and rich students. All the sites narrated by the personal reflections of my brother fulfilling his dream of presenting this great city to his nephews. One of the final drivebys was Northwestern Hospital where Sonny had spent so many harsh months being treated for leukemia. Chris was especially interested in seeing this hospital and hearing about the care which Sonny had been given. At that time he was approaching his final year of med school and needed to choose three schools for a residency. In the Fall, Match Day, a national day where all Senior year medical students are matched to one of their three choices to do a residency, was fast approaching. Chris had chosen two schools and at the time had not quite considered a third choice. Everyone was impressed by this massive hospital sitting on the edge of Chitown, especially Chris.

No one in the car asked the hard questions. Are you in remission? Will this disease need further treatment. Will you ever get stronger, maybe with a bone marrow transplant? No the typical question consisted of , "How are you feeling?" with the typical answer always being, "O.K." All the medical minds in that car but not one of us wanted to probe too much into answers we didn't want and dreaded hearing. Match Day came that Fall. For Chris, he happily accepted a residency in internal medicine at Northwestern.

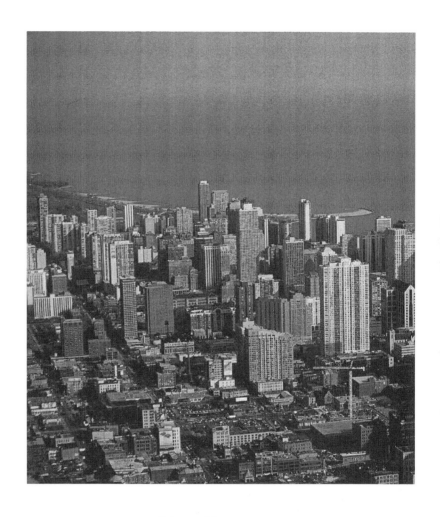

Chicago, Ill.

CHAPTER 7

SEPTEMBER

Sonny and Gail both continued to plug along and in September made a trip back to Pittsburgh to visit and reassure my mother who was living in the same Aspinwall home we grew up in but now owned by my brother, Gil. The first floor of the three story victorian had been converted to a semi apartment for my mother and my Dad where he lived until he died five years before. Gil and Ginny were gracious offering this alternative for them, instead of an assisted living apartment. Have you ever heard the song, "Feels Like Home Again" by Bonnie Raitt? It was featured in the movie, "How to Lose a Guy in Ten Days" starring Kate Hudson and Matthew McConaughey. That's exactly how I felt sitting there in our old dining room turned living area, with my mother and brothers. Sonny's playfulness shot down any prospects of talking about his future medical treatments. "Hey Chubby," my mother's nickname, "How come you never came to see me in the hospital? Oh I know you needed a crane to get you out of that chair!" My mother had an eye condition that seriously affected her vision. She couldn't really see how her once fat faced chubby boy had become thin, drawn, weakened. She could only delight in his presence, his laughter, his love.

What did we all do after visiting Mother? We went to a bar, of course! Thanks to my oldest brother , Danny, who had reserved a spot at his favorite, Bob's Garage. This place all knew Danny as well as Norm was known in the T.V. sticom, " Cheers". In fact when Danny arrived all sitting at the bar said, "Norm". Danny physics somewhat matched that of Norm's.

Bob's Garage is always decorated 360 degrees for whatever the holiday at the time. It is pretty much unmissable on the side of the road because of the amazing number of lights. They actually close down for 4 days to put up the decorations and it shows! The 4th of July red white and blue was plastered over every single wall, ceiling, and bar area. On entering the bar area Sonny just had to remark. "Did Uncle Sam throw up in this place?" The waitress came to take our order. "Hon, 4 waters lots of ice , 4 Iron Cities cold. O.K.?" "Kitten, remember Fat Misty?" Oh, I could tell a story was about to be recapped.

When Tom and I were first married, we decided to vacation with Sonny and Gail at a beach in Wildwood, New Jersey. Neither of us had excessive amounts of money so we split a hotel room at an alluring compound on the North end of town, away from the clamor of the boardwalk. It was fun to enjoy the pool that had a high diving board and the crashing ocean waves, but as the week went on we looked for a different adventure. Gail suggested riding horses on the beach. A picture immediately circumscribed my mind of a beautiful girl galloping along by the white capped, crystal blue sea, with her hair blowing behind. "Let's do it," I immediately chimed in. Not soon after the decision was made we arrived at the stables north of Cape May.

"Reality is merely an illusion, albeit a very persistent one." (Albert Einstein)

The weather was not quite the clear blue day that we see in the commercials. That day the humidity hung like a dome over a pot of steam. We all set off trotting behind the guide on our horses through the woods, and through the woods, and through the mosquitoe-infested woods for one long hour. Gail having had some equestrian training kept asking to cantor and eventually gallop. But the guide seemed oblivious to our requests leading us by a slow trot. Sonny held up the rear on his horse named Fat Misty. When we finally reached the beach the guide was quick to set us free but warned not to have the horse go any faster than a trot. Apparently the sand on the beach could harm the horse's ankles and legs. My visual image turned into more of a pony ride at a child's birthday party. All four horses were barely able to trot in the fog hung humid air on the soft sandy beach by Cape May, New Jersey. Fat Misty continued to lag last in line. On the way back the guide picked up the speed knowing we were expecting more from our adventure. Gail and Tom delighted in getting their horses to cantcr and Tom later claimed, after a few beers, that he was galloping. After we dismounted and were waiting around the stables we noticed Sonny was no where to be seen. Five minutes went by, ten minutes, fifteen minutes sent the guide into the woods to investigate. As we stood by the stables in our exhausted-bug ridden state, we witnessed Sonny finally walking out of the woods with his hat pulled down low, guiding Fat Misty by the reigns. "She got tired about half way through. I couldn't even get her to move!" The whole adventure was documented by pictures that were unfortunately lost by the film processor at the pharmacy that Tom was working at the time. None of us ever forgot about the day we rode horses on the beach!

After the bar, Sonny wanted to see some of the "sights of Pittsburgh". Gil immediatetely jumped to the chance of driving him to get a glimpse of his favorite spots in the Burgh. Gil has been a limo driver for many years and can whip through the hills and valleys that make Pittsburgh so very unique. He showed him Highland Park, Oakland, Troy Hill, Regent Square, the Strip District where Iron City Beer was first made and the Point where two rivers converge to make the mighty Ohio river. "That's where Art Rooney's home is! There's the house Dad grew up in. A new upscale shopping area's planned to be built there where the old J&L mills stood."Gil did all the talking and Sonny inaudibly listened as if it were the first time he had ever seen these sights. Sadly it was the last time he would see them. The tour ended with a trip to the top of Mt. Washington by riding up the Duquesne incline. After the pulley system asended the ominous hill, they climbed out to stand and observe the amazing sight of downtown Pittsburgh unfold before their eyes. The sun's fading dusk light cast dim shadows on the highrise buildings and bridges that stretched across the rivers. Gil was silent as they took this in together and felt a deep remorse over the finality of this experience with his brother. Sonny brought relief from the somber moment with his words, "Let's get something to eat." Gil happily agreed by adding, "How about a Primanti"s!"

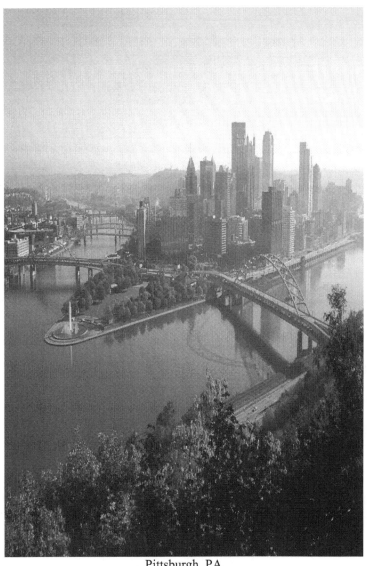

Pittsburgh, PA

Chapter 8

November
Two Phone Calls

It was all of a sudden November! For me the normal routine of working, going to the kids games, keeping up with day to day living had replaced the constant pins and needles mood that had plagued us all summer. Normalcy isn't a bad thing. As a special education teacher, a routine is the prime goal for the students. That year my students needed a consistant, structured environment. Eventhough they consisted of Autistic, Mentally Retarded, and Emotionally Disburbed children, they all had trouble learning third grade level material. It was my job to make them, "normal". In a way, I was thankful for this routine. As a family we were lost in the mundane of living rather than overtaken by the fearful reality of dieing.

One Tuesday in late November as I was assembling various things together for dinner, the phone rang. It was Sonny. "Kitten, I didn't want to tell anyone but I've been in the hospital the past few weeks. The doctor just left and told me that everything they can do has been exhausted and well I'm going ahead on to heaven, and I'll save a place up their for you. O.K.?" All this in one long sentence. All the questions and uncertainties about this disease called leukemia had just been summed up for me in one sentence! I could only react with tearful mutters of support and love. We didn't speak long, I knew he had a chain of phone calls to make. I knew that his strong faith was going to pull him through.

It is a blessing to be raised in a big family. The routine I just spoke about couldn't just be ignored or put on an unknown hold. Tom often has the saying, "Those day jobs always get in the way." The best luxury would have been to escape to Chicago and hold vigil with Gail. Luckily, my sister, Weezie, was able to clear her schedule to sustain our brother in his final month.

Another phone call came in mid December. This time I was at school. I had to take the call right outside my classroom in the hall. It was Tom's sister calling to tell me that she had a message from my mother, who was trying to reach me and didn't know my work number. With a room full of students within eye's view, I learned that Sonny had died. All I wanted to do was see him one more time. Why didn't I take off and visit! The anguish felt following was irrepressible. The principal immediately arrived and I was able to go be with my mother. As I was leaving my eye caught hold of one of my students. Jamie was an emotionally disturbed child who would rather throw his desk down to the ground than do the work I had put on top of it. On that moment he held big alligator tears along his fat rounded face and mouthed, "I'm sorry." The vision of Jamie stayed with me throughout the entire funeral.

Driving to Aspinwall, I became more attuned to supporting my mother. How awful it must be to lose a child. How could she ever handle this in her weakened, frail state. My mother had taught us how to have faith and that prayer would solve anything. But I couldn't imagine her state at this moment. Danny and Gil were at the house and they could tell I was upset. But somehow my mother got the news wrong. Sonny wasn't dead, he was in a sedated coma to offset the trauma he felt from his body slowly shutting down. A heavy weight was just lifted from my inner being. I decided in the split second "We're all going to Chicago, now!" Danny, Gil and I piled into Gil's van to make the pilgrimage and see our brother for the last time. I secretly felt I was just given a great gift.

When we arrived at the hospital late that night, Weezie met us at the door cleary dissheveled and exhausted. "I'm going! He tore off all his clothes and pulled out all his I.V.s! He was trying to escape. They had to sedate him heavily. I just need to get out of here."

So it was my turn to keep night watch with Sonny. As he slept in this state of numbness, I began to use a practice a nurse taught me many years before. It's called theraputic touch. As my hands were brushing away all the bad energies lingering within, I realized that this was in no way meant to be a cure or miraculous recovery, just something I controlled in a private moment with my brother.

Danny came to relieve me around 2a.m. Just as I was getting ready to get in the make shift bed/chair, Sonny sat up, saw us and said, "Who threw the party and didn't invite me?" My brother was back, in his right mind, with his humor, in all his glorious self. The next day Gail came as soon as she heard that Sonny was awake. She also had been struggling with her health issues and clearly looked worn down. She saw his smiling face, didn't say a word to anyone, just laid down beside him on his hospital bed. I don't know how much time passed in those moments. I just know it was the most touching display of love that I have ever seen. It was a gift to get Sonny back for all of us, if only for a short time.

Sonny was released from the hospital to go home to die in his little postage stamp community with hospice care. We had to get back to our day jobs and left Sonny to my brother Pierce and his sons Pierce Jr. and Scott. It was the week before Christmas, but time just seemed inconsequential.

However, with 4 children, I didn't have the luxury to not have Christmas. Chris, Susan, and Jeff would be coming home. The house was decorated,the gifts were wrapped, and the cookies were made. Christmas Eve on our street is very picturesque with luminar candles lit wrapping around the curves of both streets. Our cozy cape cod fits very nicely into the Christmas Currier and Ives post card with its roaring fireplace and tiffany lamps. The first year Susan came into our lives, we hosted her family to dinner on Christmas Eve. Since then it had grown to be an annual event for extended families and friends. Cooking the ham, the scalloped potatoes, the chocolate truffle, trying to form dainty hor d'ovres; provided a temporary escape from the imminent death of my brother.

Christmas Eve Mass for the children was a very popular Mass because of its convenient time of 5:00. That year it was being held in our local High School auditorium. The day wisked past because of all the needed preparations and before I knew it I was sitting with my suited-up boys and Tom ready to begin our Christmas Eve celebration with Mass. Sonny had been put in my back pocket of emotional awareness. We even got seats together in the daunting auditorium. As the opening song, "Silent Night" was played, I suddenly knew I couldn't sit there a minute longer without breaking down. Some kind of switch was turned on and tears surged in my eyes leaving me no choice but to make a quick departure. Tom and the boys were well too familiar with my emotions when in a church setting which made the exit inconsequential. At that point, I took the car to the adjacent park planning to usher in the birth of Christ from on top of the hill looking over the barren icy trees. An isoated moment of peace made its presence as time nearly came to a stop. This moment was burst by such a desperate sinking feeling that sent me immediately home to seek out some kind of sanctuary. Entering the house I bolted in just in time to catch the phone ringing. It was Danny. "Sonny died. I already called Weezie , Pierce, and Gil. He died at 5:10. You know, Karen, I called Gail just at the time he died. I felt him tugging at me so I called and he had just died. Tears poured from my eyes, just as they are now while I am writing this. I can only marvel at the astounding bond that is shared as family members. Each one of his siblings sensed Sonny's presence as he passed from this world into divine eternity.

Faith, that's what got me through the next several hours. The faith which gave me a reassurance that Sonny was now home and on this special night! Leave it to Sonny to crash a birthday party. The special door in St. Peter's Basillica are opened every 100 years. Sonny got to be one of the first ones through those doors. "Imagine the birthday cake you'll have tonight!"

All these thoughts went through my head like shooting stars in a meteor shower as I drove to pick up everyone after Mass from the make-shift church. I held onto the happenings almost selfishly, only wanting to bare the news myself. Before our guests started arriving, I privately told Tom allowing him into my grief-stricken world. We gave each other the strength we needed to proceed onto the night and decided to wait until after everyone had gone to tell the kids. In the special magic of Christmas Eve, seeing the glow of luminars lighting an endless path to somewhere unknown, I felt a peace which is to date unduplicated. After the guests had left, Susan sat down with me to give me my Christmas gift. It was a DVD featuring John Denver, my favorite singer who had died over five years before. She insisted we watch it together, on the couch. At that point my hardened persona caved and could no longer hold in my true emotions. I then realized that she knew just as all my children had been discretely given the news. One by one Tom, Chris, Jeff, Andy, and Graham joined us on the couch to listen to "Country Roads" and "Rocky Mountain High". Nothing could be heard except the music of John Denver and the frequent whimpering from tears.

Chapter 9

December
The Funeral

Christmas morning took on a whole knew light than the normal excitement of unwrapping presents. This year we experienced a new type of presence . The presence of being with each other, consoling my mother's broken heart, figuring out the details of Sonny's funeral. Danny and Gil thought strongly about having the funeral in the beloved town where he grew up, Aspinwall. This way would have allowed my mother to be present. Gail called in just as we were in the middle of this heated debate. Gail along with Sonny and Weezie had made all the funeral arangements the week before. The viewing would be in Munster on the 28th followed on the next day by the funeral mass and burial. Gail decided that the casket would only be opened for us to view before 1:00 then closed to everyone else who visited. As a compromise for Danny and Gil a memorial service was planned the next weekend for my mother and hometown friends to attend. The rest of the day seemed to disappear in quiet reflections of the days to come, while trying to remain in the Yuletide spirit.

The day after Christmas is our wedding Anniversery. "Get married the day after Christmas," my Mother would advise, " The flowers would be free." Tom and I had been married 29 years that year. We were determined to celebrate together with a cozy dinner in front of a blazing fire and a cracked open bottle of chardonnay. I was fine as the prep for all of the day's events rumbled on, until the newspaper came. There is something about seeing in print an obituary about your brother. My eye caught the heavy black headline; Aloyuis Martin Frauenheim III dies. I lost every ounce of any control that had been rallied within me. For those couple minutes, obituary in hand , I allowed myself to grieve for the loss which left

such a deep hole in my very being. Losing a
sibling is truly like losing part of yourself.
"We came into the world like brother and
brother; And now let's go hand in hand, not one
before another." -William Shakespeare

   Tom had planned the ETD at 4:00 a.m.in the
morning on the 28th. Danny and Gil's families
rented one of Danny bus companies vans so as to
all fit in one car. At 3:45 we noticed Jeff was no
where to be found. As the minutes approached
the ETD, óne could see the steam of anger rising
from Tom's head. Luckily at 3:55 Jeff came
strolling in, "Well, are you ready?" Jeff smugly
asked with a smile. He had been to his five year
High School reunion the night before. Only
snickers from Andy and Graham could be heard
as we piled into the mini van filled to capacity. It
was a frigid, icy night leaving windows that you
couldn't see out of because of the frozen ice. I
sat beside Susan in the back seat and noticed her
etching out little circles on the ice-coated
window, I imagine to get some kind of vision of
where we were headed. Susan was not a good
traveler. She hated flying and was skitish about
driving on long trips in a car. Tom was the main
driver and admitted to not feeling good. He had
all the symptons of the flu; chills, sore throat,
cold. I guess that steam coming from his head

that I mentioned earlier was in actuality a fever. He persevered along in spite of how he felt, as he has been able to do throughout his whole life. I knew it wasn't perfect but all I could feel was penetrating peace and comfort of all being together in our van on that icy cold night going to be with my brother for a final time.

Chris took over the driving around 10:00 a.m., when we got a phone call from Gil. Their rented van had broken down just before the Indiana border which we had passed 10 miles before. Tom directed the plan to turn around by finding the next exit. As Chris slowed down to look for it, we saw two cars ahead totally do a 360 on the glare ice which coated the highway. Things became markedly quiet in the car. We were unsure of the outcome of even getting to the funeral. The tow truck had just arrived at the scene when we pulled off the highway behind the broken van. The temperature at the time was -10, resulting in the driver of the tow truck allowing the lightest passengers to ride in the van while it was being towed. This is normally illegal but the alternarive would have been to let people alone on the Highway with frigid temperatures. Since most of my children filled that requirement, they proceeded to pile in the disabled van now elevated from being put on the tow truck. This parade of lightweights included Susan, who had only a look of terror in her eyes with not one word of protest. As my brothers stood in the parking lot of the garage lamenting the fact that we would not make it in time to see the open casket, I thought of Sonny shaking his head and saying, "They can't even get to my funeral on time! Dominos, patris, et felius etc." My private thoughts turned to nervous snickering which spread to our circle of problem solvers. We were all standing frigid cold in that lot laughing irrepressibly. Tom finally came to his senses and said, "Just rent a car. You can pick up the van on the way back. Just do it!"

We arrived at funeral home two hours late and to our surprise it was already full of people paying their respects. Time didn't allow us to check in at the hotel, freshen up, look presentable for this somber occasion. No, we were forced to arrive as is, looking like tired weary, sick travelers. Chris and Jeff were accustomed to looking presentable on the cusp of a dime. They lived in the disarray of dorm rooms and apartments. I always marveled at their ability to secure a well-groomed dressed appearance from the ball of clothing left on the floor. As they entered the funeral home, each sported a suit, complete with dress shirt and tie. Tom, however, did not have either the energy or the ingenuity to do anything but pull on his raincoat buttoned up close to hide the wrinkled Christmas plaid flannel he had on since the night before. It warmed me to see this poor flu-sicken man looking more like a sick Columbo than his usual neatly dressed appearance.

Eye-opening encounters happened in the following two hours! People immediately approached us with heartfelt words of condolences followed by stories of their happenstances with Sonny. Working as a Human Relations director for LTV had been a challenging job in light of the decline of steel making in the United States. Sonny was responsible for getting people jobs. This he did with great delight! Every kid in Aspinwall who needed a summer job to raise money for college got a job in the mills of J&L Steel through Sonny. Tom even worked on the coke ovens one summer during college. However, the unions got bigger and demand grew smaller causing multitudes of lay offs and the eventual shut done of J&L Steel in Pittsburgh. This took an enormous toll on my brother now needing to turn mentor and advisor to those looking for alternative work. He used every connection he could for his workers to find a replacement career for their lifelong job at the mill. For Sonny to stay employed meant him moving to Indiana to be in H.R. at the parent company LTV. We actually all thought this was simply a lame duck way of easing into retirement in a couple years. Sonny never really spoke to us about his job at LTV.

Nothing could have surprised us more than the multitudes of people from LTV grateful for knowing Sonny and becoming the benefactors of his help. One man, I remember, told me the story of calling Sonny on a Sunday morning. His wife had been seriously ill and he was admitting her to the hospital, but had questions about their coverages from work. Instead of staying on the phone to relate the red-tape involved, Sonny simply said, "I'll be right over." This man tearfully related the morning Sonny sat with him in the hospital until his wife was secure in the hospital and treatment had been started. In five short years my brother had made a lasting impact on hundreds of people by doing all he could to help each one. Nothing impressed my family more as we each took in earfulls of grateful co workers and friends.

The interim time between funeral hours gave us a chance to check-in, clean up and then proceed to Sonny and Gail's house where the neighbors had dinner waiting. They also made lasting friendships with Sonny and Gail. Sonny had been instumental in their lives first by getting one daughter a summer job at LTV and then by getting the younger daughter an interview at St Mary's Notre Dame where she attended the next fall. Again we saw Sonny's generosity at work in yet more lives.

After dinner my nephew Pierce, who like all of us was dealing with great loss, thought we should go around the room and say one thing about Uncle Sonny, as a toast to his life. One after another his neices and nephews related tales of their special relationship with Uncle Sonny. "He took me to a Chicgo Bulls game!", said Gail's sister's son Scott. "He always attended all of my son Christopher's birthday parties and gave us lots of hats!" said Michael, Gail's other nephew. "I learned all about the stock market." said Andy. Gil and Ginny's son, Adam, spoke of the many weekends he would spend hanging out at their house. One after the other voiced their heartfelt connection to Uncle Sonny. We adults stood in awe filled with surprise and gratitude that someone had made this kind of impact on our children. When the evening was over, I thought to myself, how can one person have such an impact on so many? How do you make everyone you encounter feel as though they are the most impotant to you?"   Sonny and Gail could not have children of their own but certainly left a legacy of unconditional generosity.

The next morning we woke up to a delicious day with whipped cream clouds against a midwestern blue sky. This was a sharp contrast to the cold icy ridden world we had experienced the day before. Tom admitted that he was even feeling a bit better. As I was standing in the hotel room ironing the 4 pair of kakies and dress shirts, my boys never travel pressed and ready to go, I heard Jeff say, "Maybe I can take a shift today". My semi trance response that I often find myself in while ironing was , "Oh I wish I could, you know us girls can never have success when we travel." My family erupted in immediate laughter! "I meant take over the driving since I wasn't up all night like the night before!" From that day on anything that goes on in the bathroom has been renamed, a shift.

Gail and Weezie had planned a glorious spiritual good-bye for Sonny. The songs during Mass allowed us to grieve and pray for our brother as he passed from our world into heaven.

"I will fly you up on Eagles' Wings, Make you to shine like the sun!" "Make me a channel of your peace; where there is hatred, let me so love. Where there is despair in life; only hope." These words were the saving hand to lead us from grief and provide glimpses of Sonny's eternal new home. Such fitting comforting words to engulf our senses and wipe away the tears!

A eulogy was delivered from a Co-worker at LTV who worked with him for 20 years both in Pittsburgh and Chicago. These are some of his remarks.
"A treasure is a treasure because it is wonderful unique and irreplacable. What a treasure we had in Al Frauenheim. He left his mark on all our lives in a very special way. He certainly left his mark on LTV! He was incredibly hard working and dedicated doing whatever was required to get the job done right! He was one of the most result-oriented people I've ever had the pleasure to work with—Al just liked to get things done and move on to the next challenge.

During his 35 years at LTV and J&L, Al garnered more President's and General Manger's Awards than any other employer in our history. He was the consummate team player—happy in any role he was asked to play.

There was another important constant in how Al performed his job—he was always fair and incredibly compassionate. He possessed a genuine concern about people and has touched many of our lives with his thoughtfulness and concern. Even as he waged his own heroic stand against leukemia, he was still looking out for others in his special way. I have an 18 year old nephew who is fighting cancer. Knowing this, Al arranged for us to take him to a resort in West Virginia. Not only did Al set up a wonderful weekend for this young man but in typical Al fashion, he called him each morning to make certain everything was perfect and to help in setting up the day's activities. He just loved to make people feel special."

A treasure is a treasure because it is wonderful unique and irreplacable. I know I speak for all of us in saying we will miss you dear friend—you are our treasure."

Aloysuis Martin III was buried on December 29,1999; my birthday. All of us preferred to call him Sonny. Happy new birthday, Sonny.

Epologue

Shortly after the funeral we received a birth
notice that Patrick Aloysius was born on
September 22, 2000.   What a wonderful
continuation of life for us to witness.
Chris accepted a resedency at North Western
Hospital 2000 and studied under some of the
same doctors that treated Sonny. He and Susan
spent three incredible years living in Chicago.
$ 5,000.00 was donated to Team Leukemia for
the 2002 Chicago Marathon. Thanks to Chris
and Susan, Jeff, Matt, and Craig.
Each one of Sonny's 20 nephews and neices
inherited half of his estate. Which ended up
being $10,000 each.
Gail died two years later on December 29, 2002.
Charles Aloysius Rihn was born on March 23,
2009. He is the son of Jeff and
Theresa Rihn.

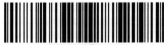

Made in the USA
Charleston, SC
30 November 2011